<u>Stallone May (M.D).</u>

HEALING with URINE THERAPY.

<u>Urotherapy For Treating;</u> *ACNE, TUBERCULOSIS, CHLOASMA/MELASMA, ECZEMA, BEES BITE, BURNS, BLISTERS, SCROFULOSIS, BRUCELLOSIS, WARTS, MALARIA, SCABIES, CONJUNCTIVITIS, GLAUCOMA, ASTHMATIC CONDITIONS, TOOTHACHES, PEPTIC ULCER.*

Disclaimer.

This book has been independently written and published strictly for informational and educational purpose(s) only. It is not intended to serve as a medical prescription of any kind.

You should endeavor to consult/visit a professional healthcare expert for appropriate counsel before embarking on any medical therapy on this book.

Table of Contents

CHAPTER ONE.

INTRODUCTION TO UROTHERAPY/URINE THERAPY.

The existence of urine is as old as creation itself. Urine is obtained from the waste products of animals and man. Urine has its special and unique features, which differentiate it from every other fluid whether obtained from man or from animals. In the early Greek and Roman, most treatments that were urine-based weren't properly documented. however, it was during the medieval Hindu-Indian era that urotherapy started gaining momentum and good relevance, in those days, this act was called Amaroli (because the people strongly believed that drinking of their urine had a good number of benefits to their health).

In ancient Europe, urine sipping prescription was documented to have originated in ancient Rome, Egypt, and Greece. After the expiration of the Roman empire, urine therapy spread to India and China, as seen in the early writings and inscriptions all over these countries.

WHAT IS URINE MADE OF?

In the kidney organ where urine is primarily produced, urine is very sterile. It is uninfected, but only becomes contaminated when it is excreted outside the body, although it is not toxically infected.

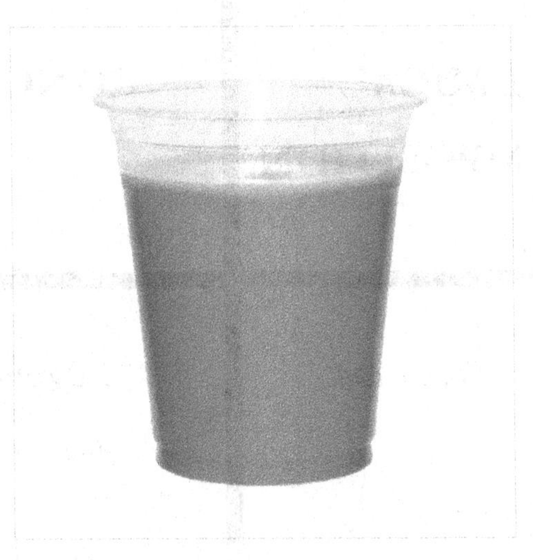

Urea is famous for its diuretic substance effect, which was discovered to be very active in treating oedema and ascites infections.

CHEMICAL COMPOSITION.	CONC.
◖ Creatinine cpd.	◖ 1.5grms per day.
◖ Electrolytes	◖ 10grms per day.
◖ Uric acid cpd.	◖ 1g per day.
◖ Organic Acids.	◖ 3grms per

day.

💧 Water	💧 90% and above.
💧 Urea	💧 25g per day

CHAPTER TWO.

CLASSIFICATION OF UROTHERAPY ADMINISTRATION.

In this section of this book, we will be discussing the various classifications of urine therapy's health benefits. This will throw more light on the under-discussed curative tendencies of your urine.

Administering urine creates the right platform for bile to be activated and absorbed into the body.

❑ <u>HORMONAL RE-ABSORPTION IN URINE THERAPY.</u>

Hormones like thyroidal, adrenal gland hormones, and other non-protein related hormones are reabsorbed into the body, when you consume your urine.

Administering urine via tropical/dermal application creates the right avenue for the hormones to be absorbed into the body. Just apply the urine on your skin and massage it gently on the skin, it will sink in through the skin's surface.

Morealso, hormonal melatonin is also a special kind of hormone that is produced

and found in the mid-stream morning urinating session. It possesses a good calming effect with a powerful anti-aging and anti-cancer characteristics.

Urine has shown to be a very effective therapeutic source of healing from allergies and skin disorders like eczema, asthma, psoriasis, rheumatism, as well as fever, as a result of the adrenal steroidal cortex hormones that are secreted.

❑ <u>URINE NUTRIENT RE-ABSORPTION & REUSE (ENZYMES AND BILE AS A CASE STUDY).</u>

Through the application or administering of urine either by orally drinking it or a massage, quite a handful of the nutritional elements like amino-acids, vitamins & hormones re-enter the body and reserve the body as vital nutrients.

❑ <u>RELATED HEALTH BENEFITS OF URINE THERAPY.</u>

Despite the talks in some quotas about the unwholesome nature of urine, its taste, and smell. Urine has quite a lot of healthy benefits;

- It helps in improving eye-sight, when properly applied.

- Urine treatment aids in the replacement of lost nutrients.

- It treats a lot of illnesses significantly when prescribed and administered correctly.

- Urine therapy boosts and improves bodily immunity, as well as supports the improvement of thyroidal health.

- Sometimes in dire situations, urine can be used as an alternative source of water. This has been proven by individuals who have traveled the desert regions of the globe illegally.

According to research, the composition of urine varies when there are traces of sickness in the body. Citing a liver blockage medical condition, which could cascade into Hepatitis, is often caused as a result of the inability of the liver to produce a reasonable quantity of bile. And as a result, makes it extremely difficult for the body's digestive system to digest fatty foods and proteins.

❑ <u>CAN SOMEONE ELSE'S URINE BE CONSUMED?</u>

In dire and rare situations where a patient is deemed too weak to pass out urine and his/her urine is required for administration, a healthy relative or person of the same sex could come in.

A female's urine is said to have a significant number of feminine hormones, as well as a male has a significant number of masculine hormones in his urine. If any of these parties continue to consume each other's urine, after a long time, such party would have traces of acting like the opposite sex.

CHAPTER THREE.

URINE THERAPY AND DISEASES.

PART I.

⅄ URINE THERAPY AND ENZYME.

Urine is well-ladened with enzymes, which is why it can be used to treat Hypertension, arteriosclerosis, pulmonary embolism, and others. The urokinase enzyme is the key enzyme that is actively involved in curative procedures. This enzyme can even be derived from urine

Urine, from studies, has been shown to be rich in urea and ammonia substances, which makes it exhibit a great deal of anti-viral, anti-bacteria, anti-septic, and purifying effects.

These healing effects is/are also felt in the skin when you happen to have a scratch or a fresh cut in your skin. For most persons, when you administer urine to the part of the body where this incident occurs, it prevents flies and immediate infection.

⚔ <u>URINE AS A DOTIXIFY AND LAXATIVE AGENT, ESPECIALLY DURING YOGA.</u>

One of the constituents of urine is salt. In yoga exercise, salt water(urine) is used in the cleaning and purification of the body from within, and this helps to eliminate or reduce the adverse effects of asthma, constipation, and even stomach ulcers. Apart from the earlier mentioned positive impact of salt water, it also helps in the removal of mucosal substances from the internal lungs and organs.

URINE THERAPY AND FACIAL ACNE.

Although Urotherapy also known as urine therapy, trado-medically has recorded some curative effects on certain skin diseases, but has not been scientifically proven to be able to treat acne-related infections.

Although urea which is one of the constituents of urine after undergoing some laboratory tests and conditioning, is one of the highly used exfoliating and moisturizing ingredients in the making of skincare-related products around the world.

⌃ <u>URINE THERAPY & SKIN-CARE.</u>

As already emphasized in the earlier parts of this book, urea is one of the most widely used skincare raw materials. Below are some of the chemical affiliations with urea;

⌛ **As A Moisturizer:** Urea has been known both herbally and scientifically as the key element in skincare products that helps increase the hydration of the skin.

⧗ **As An Emollient Agent:** Urea helps to soothe and make the skin soft. It is found in creams and some soaps.

⧗ **As A Keratolytic Agent:** This urine compound helps in loosening the skin cells, thereby aiding skin exfoliation.

⧗ **As Skin Barrier:** Urea helps to improve the barrier functionality of the skin against harmful and irritating micro-organisms.

⚔ <u>UROTHERAPY AND TUBERCULOSIS.</u>

Tuberculosis (TB) is a contagious bacteria (mycobacterium tuberculosis) infection or disease that affects the lungs and also negatively impacts the chest region, it results in heavy and painful coughing. If left unattended, it could go further to affect the spine and brain of the body.

Tuberculosis development is in different stages and forms, which include; *Primary, Latent, and Active Tuberculosis.*

<u>Symptoms Associated With Tuberculosis.</u>

Some of the symptoms include;

- Weight loss,
- Chills and fever,
- Appetite loss,
- Persistent coughing
- Coughing out blood,
- Pain in the chest and others.

How Can Tuberculosis Be Transferred?

The contagiousness of TB is closely associated with the following forms of contact;

- Kissing,
- Hands shaking,
- Sharing of contaminated sharp objects,
- Exchange of bodily fluids,

- Sharing of toilets, toothbrushes, as well as mattress covers.

Risk Factors Associated With Tuberculosis.

- A chronic smoker,
- From a friend who has tuberculosis,
- Traveling to a tuberculosis-infested area/space,
- Being a healthcare worker.

Administering Urotherapy:

Apply urine orally by drinking half a glass of the morning midstream urine on an empty stomach, very early in the morning, for a week. You can take the urine twice a day, and get it ladened with a sweetened flavor.

CHAPTER FOUR.

URINE THERAPY AND DISEASES.

PART II.

▲ UROTHERAPY AND SCROFULOSIS.

Scrofula is a bacterial disease or infection condition which is a form of tuberculosis that is found outside the lungs. It normally forms an inflammation around the neck region of the body.

Symptoms Associated With Scrofulosis.

- Fever and chills.
- Night sweats and weight loss.

<u>Administering Urine.</u>

Gently apply urine on the neck every morning and evening to wash your neck. Sometimes it is advisable that you use a child's urine. Do this for a week or two, till you get your desired result.

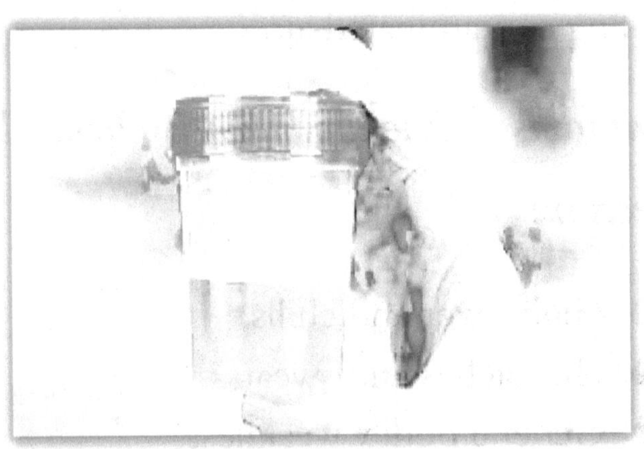

⚘ <u>UROTHERAPY AND BRUCELLOSIS.</u>

Brucellosis is a contagious bacteria infection, that is mostly transferred from animals to humans. Individuals who have brucellosis normally get this disease from the unhealthy consumption of raw dairy products, and inhaling contaminated air.

Symptoms associated with brucellosis infection:

- High fever and chills,
- Headaches and sweats,
- General bodily weakness,
- Pains in joints.

Take urine orally by drinking the morning pee for three to four days. You can as well add some flavored tea to enable a smooth drinking. Ensure to contact your healthcare expert for proper advice before you embark on this.

<u>UROTHERAPY AND LIP BLISTERS (COLD SORES).</u>

Lip blisters (Herpesviral vesicular dermatitis), also known as cold sores, are viral infections that are tiny and fluid-filled. These cold sores normally heal after fourteen to twenty-one days. Cold sores could spread from one individual to another, through very close contact, kissing, and lip fluids exchange, as possible risk factors. There happens to be no direct cure for cold sores, but the administration of prescribed anti-viral medications and creams could help manage the disease impact.

Symptoms of Cold sores:

- ◆ Swollen blisters,
- ◆ Fever, sore throat,
- ◆ Itchiness of the lip region, and
- ◆ Lip crusting,
- ◆ Headache, and some swollen aches.

WHAT CAUSES COLD SORES LIP?

Herpes Simplex Virus (HSV 1) is the virus that causes cold sores in lips.

Sharing of sharp objects with infected persons could result in cold sores on lips, and through oral sex.

Administering Urine.

Gently apply your morning urine on the affected area of the mouth, for a period of five to seven days, under the strict supervision of your healthcare expert before you do this.

<u>UROTHERAPY AND WARTS.</u>

Warts are skin tags or bumps that are seen on the skin. Warts are contagious and uncomfortable. They are generally caused by the virus called Human Papillomavirus (HPV). Wart's infection can be prevented by keeping the habit of always washing and keeping your hands clean. There are different types of warts such as; Plantar, common, flat, periungual, and filiform warts.

<u>Administering urine:</u>

Treating warts with urine is simply by administering urine on your hands, legs, or wherever the wart(s) seem to be present in any part of the body. The warts will fall off themselves.

<u>UROTHERAPY AND MALARIA.</u>

Malaria is a parasitic infection or disease that is transmitted by female Anopheles mosquitoes. Individuals who are infected by these mosquitoes fall very sick with high fever, if left untreated this illness could lead to the death of the person with the disease. The parasite is a single-cell parasite called the plasmodium, which is transmitted through the bites of mosquitoes, which in turn affects the red blood cells.

<u>Possible Signs & Symptoms Of Malaria.</u>

Some of these symptoms include; *high fever, sore throat, headache, bodily weakness, cough, abdominal pains, discomfort, and others.*

Administering Urine:

Drink your morning midstream urine, in small amounts as prescribed by your healthcare expert. Continue this practice for about seven to nine days, on an empty stomach, particularly in the morning, till you get your desired result.

CHAPTER FIVE.

URINE THERAPY AND DISEASES.

PART III.

UROTHERPAY AND SCABIES.

Scabies are generally skin diseases or infections that affect the skin, causing itchiness and sometimes scaly rashes. It is a mite infection, that lives on the skin and reproduces itself by burrowing into the skin of the body.

Scabies can be very irritating and painful, especially at night. They always infest the inner thighs, the elbows, buttocks, waist, and hands. Scabies types include Norwegian scabies, typical scabies, and nodular scabies.

To treat with urine, administer urine mixed with salt and ground roots of the autumn crocus and get the mixture rubbed all over your body every night for a period of 7 to 9 days.

⚘ UROTHERAPY AND CONJUNCTIVITIS.

Conjunctivitis is commonly known as pink eyes. It is an inflammation that is closely associated with the conjunctiva membrane. It is commonly caused by a viral infection, a bacterial, or an allergic reaction. This infection can be quite irritating and discomforting, but it doesn't negatively or greatly impact the vision of the eyes.

Administering Urine.

To treat this, you can wash your eyes with midstream early-morning urine. You can use a child's urine, which trado-medically is most effective with the best healing properties for conjunctivitis. However, in the absence of that, you can use your own urine. Wash your eyes gently with the urine every morning or you may include evenings, for about nine days.

<u>UROTHERAPY AND GLAUCOMA OF THE EYES.</u>

Glaucoma is a collection of eye conditions that harm the optical nerves of the eyes. It is this optic nerve that sends the visual information from the eyes to the brain box to enable a very clear and good vision. Glaucoma when left unattended to, could lead to blindness and can occur at whatever age, but more often rampant in elderly persons.

Some of the symptoms that is/are related to glaucoma are ***consistent redness of the eyes, blurred vision, vomiting, headaches, and Increased blinking. Also, glaucoma types*** *include angle-closure glaucoma, open-angle glaucoma, normal-tension glaucoma, and pigmentary glaucoma.*

Wash your eyes with freshly urinated mid-stream urine, for about 5 to 7days, you may stop the practice if you notice significant progress before that time. However, if it is for a growing child, you can use the mother's urine to wash the eyes.

⅄ <u>UROTHERAPY AND ASTHMATIC CONDITIONS.</u>

Asthmatic conditions are sudden and sometimes violent attacks that make breathing very challenging, due to the tightening of the airways of the lungs which become swollen and irritated and this causes the secretion of a mucosal fluid.

Symptoms associated with asthma are ***wheezing, coughing, difficulty in breathing, severe sweating, and straining of the chest muscles during breathing.***

Orally drink some urine (particularly the morning mid-stream urine). It is generally believed that a child's urine works more effectively.

⚴ <u>UROTHERAPY AND TOOTHACHES & DISEASES.</u>

Toothaches are bacteria-caused infections on the teeth, thereby leading to painful discomforts and sometimes removal of the tooth in question. Foods that are stuck in-between the teeth, and are not properly removed, sometimes even after you must have brushed your teeth. This tooth infection leads to inflammation in the gum and unwanted splitting of the tooth.

In the morning, get some urine in a glass and use it to thoroughly rinse your mouth and teeth, and pour out the urine. However, if you want to swallow the urine, you are still safe. Do this routine every morning till you get your desired results.

ALL RECOMMENDATIONS GIVEN HERE, WERE CAREFULLY RESEARCHED BY THE WRITER OF THIS BOOK. However, you **MUST** contact your health care expert for possible advice before you embark on any of the urine treatments.

CHAPTER FOUR.

URINE THERAPY AND DISEASES.

PART IV.

ʌ UROTHERAPY AND PEPTIC ULCER.

Peptic ulcers are open wounds or sores that gets to develop inside the stomach wall lining of the body. They occur also in the upper portion of the small intestine which is also known as the duodenum. Symptoms that are associated with peptic ulcer include: *heartburn, persistent pain and burning sensation in the stomach, nausea, and stomach bloating.*

Orally drink urine on a fasting or an empty stomach from the morning pee, and continue this for about seven to nine days. This has been proven to aid the quick recovery from peptic-related ulcers.

⅄ <u>UROTHERAPY AND CHLOASMA/MELASMA.</u>

Chloasma is a pregnancy skin-related disease condition. It is a "mask pregnancy", that is also known as melasma. Chloasma is caused by the over-stretching of the melanin pigment of the skin, which results in the deposit of excess melanin in the dermis and epidermis layers of the skin. Simply put, this is what causes the skin of a pregnant woman to suddenly become dark.

Get yourself to pee in a clean container in the morning, and ensure it is the mid-stream urine that you have contained in the content. Gently wash your face with the urine to remove the infections from the body, apply this for about seven to nine days.

▲ <u>UROTHERAPY AND ECZEMA.</u>

Eczema is a common skin infection or disease condition that results in the dryness and itchiness of some sections of the skin. It is a kind of dermatitis whose types include Atopic eczema, nummular eczema, contact eczema, seborrheic eczema, and others. Some possible symptoms of eczema include; skin rashness, itchiness of the skin, skin bumps, scaly or crusty skin, and others.

Apply an infant urine dermally on your skin. Do this in the morning and evenings on the region of the body where the eczema is well noticed. Continue to do this till you get a significant improvement.

⋏ <u>UROTHERAPY AND SPRAINS, DISLOCATIONS.</u>

Simply wash the dislocated or sprained sections of your body with urine, in the morning and evenings for seven days. Also, another way to apply urine on dislocated joints is to soak the urine in a clean cloth or bandage and tie it securely over the wounded area. Some people use hot urine.

⋏ <u>UROTHERAPY AND BURNS,</u>
<u>BLISTERS.</u>

A burn is a damage to the tissue of the skin, which is brought about by unsolicited heat, either from fire, chemicals, electricity, sun, or radiation. Burns types include first-degree, second-degree, and third-degree burns. The worst burn type is the third-degree burn (as it could be life-threatening most times.)

A burn-blister however is a bubble-like patch with clear liquid (called serum) on the skin. This blister kind of develops to serve as a medium for protecting the burnt area or region of the body. It helps to promote the healing of a wound.

Apply urine dermally on the skin where the burns and blisters occur. This however have no scientific backing.

⌃ <u>UROTHERAPY AND BEES BITE.</u>

Bees biting often leads to swollenness in the areas or regions of the body where the biting was felt. Here, mud needs to be used alongside the urine. Mix the urine with the mud and apply on the areas where the bee's bite is most impacted. However, in the absence of mud, crude oil can be used to mix the urine. It is pertinent to state here that you should seek the counsel of your healthcare practitioner before you go into this practice.

⋏ <u>URINE THERAPY & CANCER TREATMENT.</u>

In the mid-1960s there was a medical journal where an Indian researcher collected urine samples from both animals from both animals and man (humans). The research report stated that when the morning mid-stream urine of a human was taken, and 2-tablespoon was taken while having urine fast, for 43 days, the patient on whom this prescription was carried on, showed a significant improvement from the cancerous growth. What the urine does is to hinder significantly the further cell division of the cancerous diving cells. There was a sizeable decrease in the size of the malignant growth, but this however didn't significantly extend the lifespan of the patient.

WHY IS MEDICAL RESEARCH ON URINE THERAPY DIFFICULT?

One of the main reasons why further research on urine treatment has been hindered or relatively slow in progress over the years is due to its pungent smell and taste, particularly after the first 24hrs of its excretion.

A sample of urine when closely looked at under the lens was noticed to comprise of thousands molecular units, which makes it very difficult to isolate, and identify the most active or active elements that are curative agents.

A sample of urine when closely looked under the lens was noticed to comprise of thousands molecular units, which makes it very difficult to isolate, and identify the most active or active elements that are curative agents

<u>CONCLUSION.</u>

Urine therapeutic efficacies have been a center of discussion in biomedical research in recent times, I have already stated in the early parts of this book, suggested reasons as to why urine therapy research has been understudied over the years. Most of the urotherapeutic tendencies and history were both based on the empirical hitherto ancient knowledge and local traditional shared ideas.

THE END!!!